Making Herbal Hand Creams a~

Adapted from *Natu.*
by Norma Pasekoft

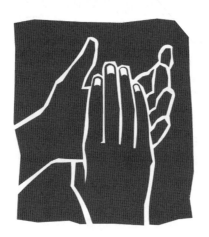

CONTENTS

Your Hardworking Hands

Just about everyone has experienced dry skin, blisters, calluses, hangnails, and red, chapped skin on their hands. Why do you think there are so many lotions, creams, and salves specially designed for hand care in the beauty products aisle of your grocery store? If you stop for a moment to think about how much your hands do for you each day, you'll appreciate the value of time spent nurturing and caring for these hardworking parts. Whether you're a mason lifting and setting rough, abrasive stone for hours on end; a gardener using shovels, rakes, and your bare hands to prepare the soil; or an office worker handling sheafs of paper all day long, your hands are likely to be dry, work-worn, and in need of some soothing relief from creams and salves.

Which lotions and creams are the best? The choice is yours. You might decide that at work you want a hand emollient that dries quickly and has no fragrance. At home you may opt for a thicker cream formula, one that you can wear all night with cotton gloves. If your hands are severely chapped and the skin is splitting, you'll want some heavy-duty salve to heal and soothe the cracked skin. And as you grow older, you'll want to use gentle, skin-nourishing lotions and creams every day to slow the effects of time.

Evaluating Commercial Products

Chances are that you won't always have the time or energy to make your own hand creams and salves. For health's sake, it's important to be an informed consumer. These are some of the ingredients to know.

Allantoin

Allantoin is a substance that is soothing to the skin. It stimulates healthy tissue formation and healing of wounds, as well as removing the scales and crusting of dead skin cells. Allantoin has a softening effect on keratin, the protein that is so abundant in the surface cells of the skin, by allowing water to be replenished in the keratin layer. This ingredient is naturally found in the herbs aloe vera, comfrey, and bearberry.

Fresh from the Farm

Hand salves and creams have probably been around since the first peoples discovered bear grease. Many nineteenth-century hand products from the agricultural communities came with names like Absorbine Veterinary Liniment, Bag Balm, Corn Huskers Lotion, and White Cloverine Salve. Farmers began to try these products, on the theory that "what's good for the horse is good for his owner."

One product, B and O'R Hand Lotion, conceived and produced by Vermont pharmacists Beauchamp and O'Rourke, was devised to cope with the industrial revolution. It was intended to protect ironworkers' hands from the temperature extremes of blast furnaces and the bitter Vermont cold. Witch hazel, camphor, soap liniment, glycerin, bay rum, rose water, and mutton tallow are some of the ingredients. Sadly, this product is no longer available.

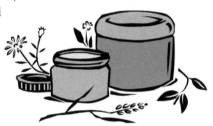

Beneficial Herbs

There are numerous beneficial herbs for hand creams and ointment recipes including aloe, calendula, chickweed, comfrey, viola or garden pansy, plantain, red clover, St.-John's-wort, and yarrow. Many are used as ingredients in commercial hand-care products.

Dead Sea Salt Extract

Dead Sea salt extract is full of vitamins and minerals and naturally increases the skin's ability to retain moisture. It is an ingredient in some high-end cream moisturizers.

Glycerin

Glycerin is a substance that attracts water but is not easily absorbed, so it will remain on the upper layers of the skin. If 100 percent glycerin is applied as a humectant, it may draw additional moisture from already dry skin. However, since the concentration of glycerin in creams and lotions is usually never more than 50 percent, glycerin can be considered a beneficial ingredient because it improves a cream's spreadability. Glycerin and rose water make a classic formulation that has been used safely for years.

Jojoba

Jojoba extract, commonly known simply as jojoba (pronounced ho-ho-ba), is similar to human sebum, the skin's natural restorative fluid. It helps to restore the skin and softens and conditions all skin types. Jojoba is cold-pressed and filtered from the seeds of a desert shrub that is cultivated in dry regions of the world, such as Israel and the Sonoran desert regions of the United States and Mexico.

Jojoba extract is an unusual wax ester with antioxidant and light emollient properties. It rarely turns rancid and does not break down under high temperatures or pressure. Jojoba became an important ingredient for the natural-cosmetics industry when it was discovered to imitate the properties of spermaceti oil — a white, crystalline, solid wax from the head of the sperm whale. Spermaceti oil was once used extensively in cosmetics, but has since been banned as a measure of protection for whales. Cetyl alcohol, a form of synthetic spermaceti oil, is an alternative to jojoba, but it can sometimes cause allergic skin reactions.

Lactic Acid

Lactic acid is a natural element of human skin. It is one of the alpha-hydroxy acids that have excellent humectant properties, attracting and retaining moisture. It also helps to maintain the acid balance of the skin.

Lanolin

Lanolin is a fatlike substance produced by oil glands in sheep and obtained from sheep's wool. It can soften dry, chapped, or cracked skin but is also known to cause some allergic sensitivities (approximately 5 percent of the population is allergic to lanolin).

Barrier Oils

Animal, vegetable, and mineral oils help to seal in moisture by forming a slick barrier on the surface of the skin. Mineral oil can be allergenic and clog the skin's pores. Petroleum jelly (petrolatum) is thick and greasy, leaves a heavy film on the skin, and can stain clothing, but it does form an effective water and environmental barrier.

Natural oils that are safe and frequently used for skin treatments include those of sweet almond, apricot kernel, avocado, olive, quince, sesame, sunflower seed, and wheat germ.

Urea

Urea is most often used as a moisturizer in a non-oily base, although it can also function as a preservative. A white, crystalline, water-soluble compound, it is a water-loving (hydrophilic) ingredient. Urea is the end product of both animal and human protein metabolism. If you are allergic to ammonia, you may be allergic to urea in cosmetics.

Preservatives

It would be much simpler if no preservatives were needed in cosmetics, but unless we plan to store all skin products forever in the refrigerator, we have to accept this necessity.

There are two classes of preservatives in beauty aids: antimicrobial agents and antioxidants. Antimicrobial agents, such as alcohol and essential oils, retard the growth of microbacteria and fungi.

Antioxidants, such as vitamins A, C, and E and carotene, block oxidation, are free-radical scavengers, and inhibit the destruction of fats and oils.

The FDA requires that the concentration of preservatives in a cosmetic product be sufficiently high to inhibit the growth of microorganisms during its use by the consumer. Without preservatives, a cream or lotion would last only 8 to 14 days (if refrigerated, about 4 weeks). With commercial preservatives, products can last 2 to 3 years.

Alcohol, essential oils, and vitamins A and E are a few natural preservatives. However, they can be expensive and volatile, evaporate when uncovered, and sometimes cause skin reddening and dermatitis. Natural-cosmetic companies tend to use the least offensive chemical preservatives available to them, such as urea and methyl parabens.

In general, many preservatives are cellular toxins, and I recommend making and using your own fresh, natural cosmetics when possible.

Recipes for Silky-Smooth Hands

Tired of rough, dry skin on your hands? Ready for a change? For smooth, soft hands, nothing beats these luxurious treatments. Try either one for the best-feeling hands you've ever had.

QUICK-AND-EASY HAND-SMOOTHING LOTION

This simple recipe is easy to make and brings great results.

> 1 tablespoon (15 ml) glycerin
> 1 tablespoon (15 ml) rose water
> 1 tablespoon (15 ml) nondistilled witch hazel extract
> 3 tablespoons (45 ml) honey

To make:

1. Blend and shake well.

2. Store in the refrigerator

To use: Pour a small amount into the palms of your hands and gently massage into your hands and fingers.

LEMONADE HANDS

This is a simple recipe that offers great results in improving the texture of your skin, shared with us by a lovely grandmother from Chile. Her hands belie her age and she confided that she has used this recipe every day for years. It smoothes the skin and acts as a mild exfoliant.

> 1   **tablespoon (15 ml) granulated sugar**
> **Fresh lemon juice to make a paste**

To make:

1. Pour the sugar in the palm of your hand.

2. Squeeze enough juice from a fresh lemon wedge to make a paste.

To use:

1. Rub your hands together in a rotary motion, either clockwise or counterclockwise. At first, the sensation will be that of a gritty, rough surface.

2. Continue rubbing. The heat of your hands will melt the sugar to become a candy glaze.

3. Work this glaze up and over each finger and over the back of each hand. Really rub your hands. Picture yourself as Lady Macbeth as she says, "Out, damned spot! out, I say."

4. Leave the glaze on your hands for 5 minutes.

5. Rinse with warm water. Pat your hands totally dry with a soft paper towel.

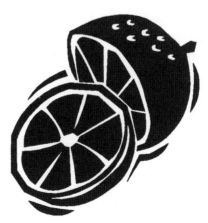

Curing Brittle, Split Nails, and Cuticles

The medical term for this problem (yes, there is a medical term) is *onychorrhexis*, splitting and brittleness of the nails. The exact causes of this condition are not known. When hands are frequently in hot water and in contact with harsh soaps, detergents, or other irritating substances, nails take the punishment. Frequent use of polish remover, which dries out the nail bed, is another common culprit.

Here's the explanation. When hands are immersed in water, the nail cells swell. Then when the nails dry, the cells shrink. With repeated swelling and shrinking, the nail will eventually split. Contrary to current opinion, the problem is not due to lack of protein, gelatin, calcium, or vitamins. There is not much calcium in the nail; its hardness is due to its special protein bonds. Extra protein or gelatin in the diet will not make our nails harder.

The best way to prevent fingernails from splitting is to keep your hands away from hot water, drying soaps, and detergents. Apply nail oil or cream often. Wear waterproof gloves for wet tasks. Cotton-lined gloves or a separate pair of cotton gloves inside rubber or vinyl gloves may offer the most protection. There are hypoallergenic gloves available now for those sensitive to latex; they are made from a material called nitrile, which resists bleach and household solvents. If these methods fail, what follows are some easy remedies to help brittle nails.

HORSETAIL NAIL CREAM

Adapted from *The Herbal Home Spa,* by Greta Breedlove (Storey Publishing, 1998)

This cream is especially good for nourishing and protecting the nails. Horsetail, although often considered a weed, is an amazing plant that has been around since the time of the dinosaurs. It is high in silica, which is found in healthy hair and nails. Make this recipe in the spring, when horsetail is in bloom. Get out your plant identification books and go out and gather it yourself. In a pinch, you can use dried horsetail. Benzoin gum resin is great for the nail bed and cuticles, conditioning where you need it most. These make great gifts.

1	cup (250 ml) fresh or ½ cup (125 ml) dried horsetail
1¼	cups (300 ml) olive oil
2	tablespoons (30 ml) beeswax
10	drops vitamin E oil
5	drops benzoin gum resin
30	¼-ounce (7 g) containers with lids

To make:

1. Place the fresh horsetail herb on a towel and allow it to wilt overnight.

2. In the top part of a double boiler, warm the horsetail in olive oil over low heat for 3 hours.

3. Grate the beeswax.

4. Strain the plant material out of the oil completely, then pour the oil back into the double boiler. Add the grated beeswax.

5. Heat the mixture until the beeswax melts completely, then remove from heat.

6. Quickly add the vitamin E oil and benzoin gum resin.

7. Pour into dainty ¼-ounce (7 g) containers or jars. Label and date.

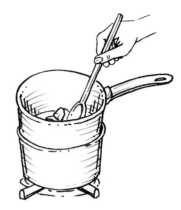

To use a double boiler, fill the bottom pot with an inch or two of water. Place over heat and set the upper pot on top. Ues the upper half for cooking — as steam rises from the lower pot, ingredients in the upper pot will warm slowly and without undue exposure to heat.

To use:

1. Use a cotton swab to dab the cream on the nail and around the cuticle of each finger.

2. Systematically massage the cream into the nail and around the cuticle of each finger.

3. Use daily and watch your fingernails shine.

MAKES THIRTY ¼-OUNCE (7 G) CONTAINERS

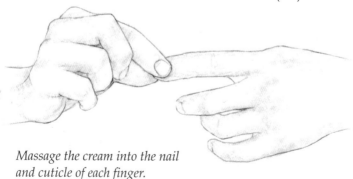

Massage the cream into the nail and cuticle of each finger.

SOOTHING NAIL AND CUTICLE OIL

Treat your nails to a warm, relaxing oil bath at least twice a week. Almond oil is a good base moisturizer for brittle or split nails. You can add the essential oils of sage, chamomile, lavender, or vanilla-like benzoin as helpful agents against any fungal infections or bacteria that might be hiding around the cuticles and under the nails. These oils also add a bit of aromatherapy to enhance your mood.

4	tablespoons (60 ml) pure sweet almond oil
20–25	drops of your choice of essential oil of sage, chamomile, lavender, or benzoin
1	vitamin E capsule (400 IU)

To make:

1. Pour the almond oil into a small bottle and add the essential oil of your choice.

2. Pierce a vitamin E capsule and squeeze it into the mixture. Shake thoroughly.

3. Label the bottle with the contents and the date.

To use:

1. When you are ready to use the blended oil, warm the bottle by setting it in a bowl of hot water for a few minutes.

2. Soak your nails in the blended oil for 10 minutes.

3. Sleep with cotton gloves on, or wrap your hands in plastic wrap covered with a towel for at least 30 minutes for extra benefit.

Caution: Lavender essential oil is not recommended for those in the first trimester of pregnancy or for those who have very low blood pressure.

Almond Joy

Eat six raw almonds every day to relieve splitting of the fingernails. Linoleic acid, an essential fatty acid (EFA), is one of the important constituents of almonds. Among other benefits, EFAs help lubricate the body's cells, which can help soften brittle fingernails.

Moisturizers for Dry Hands

If you want smoother, more pliable skin on your hands, get in the habit of using protective hand and nail creams. These creams help the skin retain moisture by adding to the natural, water-resistant (lipid) barrier between you and the environment. Soaps and detergents constantly erode this barrier. When applied to slightly damp skin, emollient creams, lotions, and ointments slow evaporation and hold on to vital moisture.

To increase skin moisture and soothe dry skin, protect yourself from skin-drying agents and use moisturizers frequently. Following are some home tips for improving humidity and moisture in skin and hands:

- Leave toilet lids up. (Don't laugh!)
- Store about 1 inch (3 cm) of water in the bathtub.
- Let aquarium fish be your pets.
- Buy a cool-mist humidifier for the bedroom.
- Wash with a mild, unscented, superfatted soap. Harsh soaps strip away natural oils and perfumed soaps contain alcohol, which is drying. Use lukewarm water and be brief. Hot water deprives the hands of moisture.
- Blot hands dry. Vigorous rubbing creates tiny tears in fragile skin. Keep a bottle of moisturizer near the sink and use it often. Apply a moisturizer each time your hands are in water. Spread the cream over slightly moist skin. Have small containers of moisturizer to carry with you away from home.
- Drink plenty of bottled water and fresh fruit juice.
- Before going outdoors, apply a sunscreen with a sun protection factor (SPF) of at least 15 to your hands.
- Protect hands with the appropriate gloves when doing wet work.

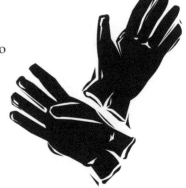

KITCHEN CABINET HAND LOTION

This is a great recipe to keep on hand at all times. Try setting out a small, travel-size container near every sink, and encourage your family to use it on their hands after washing up.

> **2 teaspoons (10 ml) cod-liver oil**
> **2 tablespoons (30 ml) castor oil**
> **2 soy lecithin capsules, pierced and squeezed**
> **1 natural vitamin E capsule, pierced and squeezed**
> **1 tablespoon (15 ml) unflavored gelatin**
> **¼ cup (60 ml) cold water**
> **¾ cup (180 ml) boiling water**

To make:

1. In a blender, combine the cod-liver oil, castor oil, contents of the lecithin capsules, and contents of the vitamin E capsule.

2. Prepare the gelatin by dissolving it in the cold water.

3. Add the boiling water to the gelatin mixture. Stir until dissolved, then cool to room temperature.

4. Add ½ cup (125 ml) of the gelatin mixture to the blender. Blend thoroughly and add only enough water to achieve the consistency of a lotion.

5. Pour into a bottle and store in the refrigerator.

To use:

Use for dry or chapped hands.

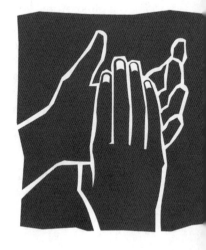

PERFECT MOISTURIZING HAND CREAM

Thanks to Rosemary Gladstar and Sage Mountain Herbs for sharing this recipe.

The proportions of this cream are about 1 part oil base to 1 part water, essential oils, and vitamins. In the oil-base ingredients, the proportions should be approximately 2 parts liquid oil to 1 part solids. Tap water is not recommended in the water ingredient because it can sometimes introduce bacteria to your cream that results in the growth of mold. If using aloe vera, the cream will be more dense but very moisturizing.

Oil-Base Ingredients

¾   cup (180 ml) apricot oil and/or sweet almond oil
½   cup (125 ml) coconut oil and/or cocoa butter
1   teaspoon (5 ml) anhydrous lanolin
½   ounce (15 g) grated beeswax

Water, Essential Oils, and Vitamins

⅔   cup (150 ml) distilled water, rose water, or orange flower water
⅓   cup (75 ml) aloe vera gel
     A few drops of the essential oil of your choice
     Vitamins A and E (optional)

To make:

1. Heat the oil-base ingredients over low heat in a double boiler until all are melted. Stir gently to mix well.

2. Pour the oil mixture into a glass measuring cup and cool to room temperature. The mixture should become thick, creamy, semisolid, and cream-colored. When completely cooled, you are ready for the next step.

3. Place the water, aloe, essential oil, and vitamins in a blender. Turn blender on the highest speed. In a slow, thin drizzle, pour the oil-base mixture into the center hole of the blender.

4. When most of the oil-base mixture has been added and the cream resembles a butter-cream frosting (you may not need to use all of the oil-base mixture), turn off the blender. Do not overbeat. The cream should be rich and thick and continue to thicken as it sets up.

5. Pour into cream jars, label, date, and store in a cool place.

To use:

Use as needed.

HAPPY-HANDS HAND CREAM

Excerpted from *The Herbal Home Spa,* by Greta Breedlove (Storey Publishing, 1998)

Everyone loves this cream, but it is especially good for dry skin. Because of spoilage problems due to rancidity, unused jars of cream must be refrigerated. Package the cream in containers that are opaque or dark to protect them from the destabilizing effects of light. I keep one cream out on my vanity and the rest take up space in my refrigerator.

Note: *The proportions in this recipe are designed for success when combined in a standard kitchen blender; a food processor will not work.*

⅓	cup (75 ml) grapeseed oil
⅓	cup (75 ml) olive oil
⅓	cup (75 ml) coconut oil
1	tablespoon (15 ml) zinc oxide paste
1	teaspoon (5 ml) cocoa butter
1	tablespoon (15 ml) beeswax
⅓	cup (75 ml) orange blossom water
⅓	cup (75 ml) distilled water
⅓	cup (75 ml) aloe vera gel
20	drops vitamin E oil
5	drops essential oil of orange blossom
5	drops essential oil of frankincense

To make:

1. In a double boiler, melt the grapeseed, olive, and coconut oils; zinc oxide paste; cocoa butter; and beeswax.

2. Once the beeswax is melted, pour the oil mixture into a glass measuring cup, preferably one with a spout.

3. Let cool to room temperature for approximately 1 hour.

4. Combine the orange blossom and distilled waters, aloe vera gel, and the vitamin E and essential oils in the blender and turn to the highest speed for a minute or two.

5. While the blender is still going, slowly drizzle the cooled oils into the vortex of the waters.

6. Listen to the blender; when it chokes, the water and oil have combined. Turn off the blender.

7. Pour cream into jars. Label, date, and store in the refrigerator.

MAKES 15 1-OUNCE (25 G) JARS

AUBREY'S OLDE ENGLISH
LYME-GINSENG MEN'S HAND CREAM

Here is a pungent, heavy-duty hand cream for hardworking hands. It was created just for Natural Hand Care *by Aubrey Hampton, an herbalist and cosmetic chemist. (You may have seen or tried some of his hair-, skin-, and body-care products under the trade name of Aubrey Organics.) The cream serves as a protective coating and with regular use will improve dry, chapped, and red hands. Although there are 14 ingredients, the recipe is easy to prepare.*

1	package (10.5 ounces, or 325 ml) "silken" tofu
½	cup (125 ml) organic aloe vera gel
1	tablespoon (15 ml) citrus seed extract
2	tablespoons (30 ml) evening primrose oil
3	tablespoons (45 ml) glycerin
3	tablespoons (45 ml) shea butter
2	tablespoons (30 ml) 100-proof grain alcohol or vodka
12	drops Siberian ginseng tonic (available from Gaia Herbs)
2	drops essential oil of ginger
8	drops essential oil of lemongrass
8	drops essential oil of lemon
2	tablespoons (30 ml) essential oil of lime
6	drops essential oil of grapefruit
1	tablespoon (15 ml) almond oil

To make:

1. Place the tofu in a food blender. Add the aloe vera, citrus seed extract, evening primrose oil, and glycerin. Blend until smooth.

2. Melt the shea butter and add it to the blender ingredients.

3. Add the alcohol; Siberian ginseng tonic; essential oils of ginger, lemongrass, lemon, lime, and grapefruit; and the almond oil. Blend until the mixture becomes smooth.

4. Pour into clean lotion bottles, label, date, and refrigerate, where it will keep for up to 3 weeks.

To use:

Use as needed. When you first apply it, the lemon-lime fragrance will be strong and there will be a bit of a sticky, clingy feeling. In a few moments, the aroma dissipates and the sticky feeling is gone.

TOUGH HANDS LOTION

Adapted from *Bodycare Just for Men*, by Jim Long (Storey Publishing, 1999)

This is a good hand lotion to use during the day.

2	tablespoons castor oil
1	tablespoon wheat germ oil
2½	teaspoons beeswax shavings
1	teaspoon vitamin E oil, 1,000 IU or more
10	drops jojoba oil
½	teaspoon lecithin
15	drops grapefruit seed extract
4	drops chamomile essential oil
5	drops myrrh-infused essential oil
5	drops tea tree oil
8	drops lavender essential oil

To make:

1. Combine the castor oil, wheat germ oil, and beeswax in a microwave-safe bowl. Dampen a paper towel and drape over the top of the bowl. Heat in a microwave on low in 20-second increments, stirring in between, until the beeswax is melted.

2. Stir or whisk well, then add the remaining ingredients and mix well again. Continue whisking until the mixture begins to harden to a salvelike consistency. Scrape into a small container and set aside until completely cooled. The mixture should now be heavier than a lotion but a little lighter than a salve.

To use:

Scoop out a fingerful of the mixture and place it in the palm of your hand. Massage this cream briskly all over your hands, rubbing it in well. This treatment is soothing, and if used on a regular basis, it will soften the skin so that healing can take place.

HONEY OINTMENT

This easy-to-make ointment will heal and rehydrate hands and arms. Honey is antibacterial and works as a humectant, meaning that it pulls moisture to the skin. It's also wonderful to smooth on nicks, bruises, and minor burns to encourage healing.

1 ounce (30 g) beeswax
1 cup (250 ml) olive, almond, or apricot oil
⅓ cup (75 ml) honey
Up to 60 drops (3 ml) essential oils of rose geranium, lavender, or bergamot (optional)

To make:

1. In a double boiler, melt the beeswax. Stir periodically to facilitate melting. This process should take approximately 10 minutes.

2. Add the oil to the melted beeswax. Stir until thoroughly blended.

3. Remove from heat and let cool slightly. Add honey and stir until incorporated. If desired, add essential oils now.

4. Pour into jars. Wait until room temperature to cap. Label and date. Jars can be stored at room temperature.

To use:

Smooth on affected areas.

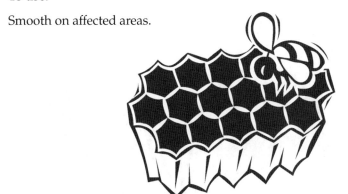

Softening and Smoothing Calluses

As we age, we have less cushioning tissue than normal and are thus more susceptible to calluses. One particular type of callus is often found on the palms of people who use assistive walking devices such as canes and walkers. The roughening and thickening is caused by the constant pressure and friction on the palm. Blisters may precede calluses. This change in the outside surface of the skin can cause tenderness in the tissues beneath.

GREEN RUB

This mild abrasive wash will gently smooth calluses from the palms.

> **1–2 tablespoons (15–30 ml) cornmeal**
> **1 tablespoon (15 ml) fresh mashed avocado or avocado oil**

To make:

Mix both ingredients in a bowl until they form a meal-like mixture.

To use:

1. Place the mixture in the palm of your hand. Rub both hands together and work the gritty and emollient meal into the calluses and up and around the fingers.

2. Repeat once or twice a week.

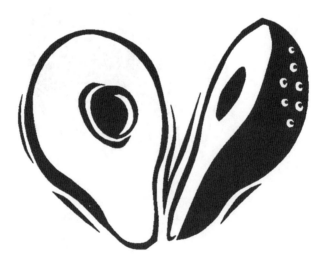

OLIVE-OIL SOFTENING SOAK

Adapted from *The Herbal Home Spa,* by Greta Breedlove (Storey Publishing, 1998)

This soak is composed of olive oil infused with sage, horsetail, and red clover. It is helpful for both brittle nails and calluses. This recipe makes enough for both hands and feet, but you can make a smaller batch for just your hands if you wish.

3	ounces (85 g) fresh sage
3	ounces (85 g) fresh red clover
2	cups (500 ml) olive oil
3	ounces (85 g) fresh horsetail
5	drops vitamin E oil
5	drops tincture of benzoin
1	16-ounce (454 g) bottle, or two 8-ounce (227 g) bottles

To make:

1. Gather the fresh herbs and lay them on a paper towel to wilt overnight. (This allows excess water in the plants to evaporate, thereby protecting your oil from contamination.)

2. The next day, combine the olive oil and wilted herb in the top part of a double boiler. Simmer on low for 4 hours.

3. Strain out the plant material, reserving the oil.

4. Add the vitamin E oil and the essential oil to this mixture.

5. Allow to cool, then bottle.

To use:

1. Pour 1 cup (250 ml) of the oil into a basin filled with warm water.

2. Immerse your hands (or feet) in the water and relax for 10 minutes. Gently massage your hands (or rub your feet) together every few minutes.

3. Remove your hands (or feet) from the water and pat dry.

Caring for Chapped, Cracked, Rough Fingertips and Palms

There are various opinions about the causes of chapped skin. The most logical explanation is overexposure of the hands to cold weather or low dew points (humidity). Another cause of chapping is repeated washing of the hands with harsh detergents. This not only chaps the hands but also allows fissuring so that contact irritants can gain entrance to the skin. Dry, chapped skin can also be one of the first signs of a vitamin A deficiency.

The most obvious remedy for chapped, cracked hands is moisturizer — and lots of it! There are several recipes listed below. However, you also want to find out why your hands are becoming so dry and chapped. If constant washing or overexposure is necessary given your job or living circumstances, moisturizer may be your only hope (although you should certainly wear gloves whenever possible). However, it may be that you suffer from a vitamin deficiency or you haven't been caring for your hands, in which case you should take preventive measures to guard against painfully cracked hands.

Vitamin Therapy

One of the first signs of a vitamin A deficiency may be continually dry or chapped hands. Are foods rich in vitamin A, such as carrots, sweet potatoes, and tomatoes, lacking in your diet? Do you have sandpaper skin or "gooseflesh" on the outer sides of your arms and legs that does not go away? If you have these bumps on your thighs, check with your healthcare provider about the possibility of taking daily vitamin A supplements.

If you have been on a stringent diet and eliminated most fats from your menu, you may also be lacking in vitamin E. Add 2 tablespoons (30 ml) of wheat germ or an unsaturated oil like corn oil — both of which are rich in vitamin E — to your daily diet. Once your skin returns to its soft, lovable self, you can gradually reduce the amount of oil or wheat germ.

SPECIAL WASH FOR CHAPPED HANDS

This is a gentle cleanser that should not be irritating to the skin. If you repeat this regimen day and night several times a week, your chapped hands will become a thing of the past.

(The cornmeal accomplishes by a gentle abrasive action what a harsh soap does by chemical action. The cornmeal, however, does not draw all the moisture away from the important lower layers of the skin.)

1	small cucumber
½	tablespoon (8 ml) honey
	Warm water
	Mild soap — fine castile, Dove, or Neutrogena
1	tablespoon (15 ml) cornmeal

To make:

1. Peel the cucumber and remove the seeds, then blend or juice the vegetable for a few seconds. Mix with the honey and set aside in a small bowl.

2. Make a paste by mixing the warm water, soap, and cornmeal.

To use:

1. Wash your hands thoroughly with the cornmeal paste. Then rinse hands well in clean, warm (not hot) water. This helps to remove flaking skin cells and any soluble environmental pollutants.

2. While your hands are damp, apply the cucumber juice and honey mixture. Have someone help you wrap your hands in plastic wrap or insert them in large, zip-seal plastic bags. Cover with a towel, then relax as long as possible.

3. Rinse and dry hands. Apply moisture cream. If you've done this at night, wear loose-fitting cotton gloves to bed. (Be sure to wash the gloves regularly.)

4. Repeat this cornmeal wash daily (and repeat as often as you can for badly chapped hands). In cold weather, substitute a *cold*-water rinse in the morning to acclimate the hands to cooler conditions. Pat dry and then massage in a moisturizing cream.

CHATHAM CHAP CREAM

Shared by herbalist Sandy Collingwood of Cape Cod, Massachusetts

This is a two-step recipe that involves first preparing an infused oil and then using the oil to prepare the cream. It's a wonderfully soothing moisturizer for chapped skin.

Step 1: The Herb Oil

1	ounce (30 g) dried lavender blossoms
1	ounce (30 g) dried comfrey leaf
1	ounce (30 g) dried chamomile flowers
1	ounce (30 g) dried calendula flowers
1	ounce (30 g) dried goldenseal leaf or Oregon grape root
	Almond oil or olive oil to cover

Step 2: The Cream

½	ounce (15 g) beeswax
⅔	cup (150 ml) infused herb oil (from Step 1)
⅓	cup (75 ml) coconut oil
¾	cup (180 ml) distilled water
¼	cup (60 ml) fresh aloe gel (or aloe extract with natural gum)
	Contents of two 400 IU vitamin E capsules

To make oil:

1. Place all five dried herbs in a large jar, cover with almond or olive oil, and seal. Place in a sunny window for 2 to 3 weeks.

2. Strain twice through cheesecloth and pour into a clean jar.

3. Seal and label until ready to make the cream. Store in a cool place.

To make cream:

1. Gently melt the beeswax in the top part of a double boiler. Add the prepared herb oil and the coconut oil. Stirring constantly, heat just enough to liquefy.

2. Pour this mixture into a glass measuring cup and cool to room temperature (10 to 20 minutes).

3. In a blender, combine the distilled water and aloe gel. Blend until it becomes thick.

4. Add the cooled oil and beeswax mixture to the aloe water. Blend in short pulses. If the beeswax is too warm, it will separate. If this happens, pour off the water and let cool until you can try again.

5. Add the contents of two vitamin E capsules. Blend. Pour into eight 2-ounce (60 g) jars with lids. Label and date the cream. Keep refrigerated.

Note: Goldenseal is now considered an endangered plant. If you purchase this herb, ask your supplier to verify that it was obtained responsibly.

Makes eight 2-ounce (60 g) jars

HONEY PASTE

Adapted from *The Herbal Home Spa,* by Greta Breedlove (Storey Publishing, 1998)

This formula is excellent for softening the most abused hands. It contains ingredients that are emollient and exfoliating at the same time, thus working to remove dry skin while softening the new skin. This recipe can also be used on the feet. It is best applied at bedtime, covered with gloves made of natural fiber, and then left on to work all night.

1 tablespoon (15 ml) almonds, coarsely ground
1 tablespoon (15 ml) oatmeal, coarsely ground
1 tablespoon (15 ml) zinc oxide paste
1 egg yolk
1 tablespoon (15 ml) honey
1 pair soft kid or cotton gloves

To make:

In a bowl, combine the ground almonds and oatmeal with the zinc oxide paste, egg yolk, and honey, stirring well.

To use:

1. Rub the paste into your hands.

2. Recruit someone to help you put on natural-fiber gloves over your paste-covered hands.

3. Go to sleep for the night, allowing the paste to work its magic. *Note:* You may not want to sleep on your best sheets and bedding if you are concerned about dripping or staining.

4. In the morning, remove the gloves, rinse your hands with cool water, pat dry, and feel the softness.

Makes enough for 1 treatment

PARAFFIN HAND BATH

Paraffin is a waxy substance that holds in heat. This causes the pores to open and allows moisturizers and healing herbs to penetrate the skin. After this treatment, your hands will feel soft, less stiff, and look great.

4 ounces (115 g, or 1 block) paraffin wax
1 ounce (30 ml) olive, almond, or avocado oil
   Olive oil (enough to grease a pan)
20 drops (1 ml) essential oil of chamomile, lemon, or
   geranium (optional)
   A few drops of St.-John's-wort or carrot seed oil, enough to
   coat your hands

To make:

1. Gently heat the paraffin, the olive, almond, or avocado oil, and the essential oil in the top part of a double boiler until the paraffin has melted. (Never heat wax directly over an open flame or burner, and never leave wax unattended.)

2. Lightly grease a 10-inch (25 cm) pie plate or a large glass or ceramic casserole with olive oil (the oil coating will make it easier to clean the pan later). The vessel should be large enough to accommodate your hand.

3. Carefully pour the melted oil and paraffin mixture into the pie plate or casserole. When a thin skin forms on the surface of the wax, the temperature should be right for dipping the hands. Test the wax mixture for temperature comfort with a drop of the wax on the inside of your wrist.

To use:

1. While waiting for the mix to cool, wash your hands and pat dry. Completely coat your fingers and hands with St.-John's-wort oil or carrot seed oil.

2. Dip each hand repeatedly into the melted paraffin mixture, to build up the wax layers. Be sure to include the thumb. The heat and oil will penetrate the muscles and tendons and help relieve stiffness and pain, as well as hydrate the skin.

3. Put each hand into a zip-seal plastic bag. You may need someone to help you if you are doing both hands. Cover both hands with a towel and relax for 15 to 20 minutes.

4. When the time is up, keep your hand in the plastic bag as you peel away the paraffin to catch all the pieces of wax. Peel away the wax (one hand at a time) by grasping the hand covered with paraffin above the wrist and pulling down — the wax should come off in large pieces. (If you've coated both hands, you'll need help with this step!)

5. Massage and gently stretch your hands.

ALMOND, COMFREY, AND HONEY SOOTHING OINTMENT

Here is a recipe from the Middle Ages for painfully cracked hands. Almonds are known for their mildness and softening action on the skin. Comfrey, also called bruisewort or knitbone, has been cultivated in gardens for centuries for the wound-healing qualities of the root and leaves. Allantoin, one of the constituents of comfrey, encourages healthy skin regrowth by stimulating cells, and also relieves itching.

1	**ounce (30 g) ground almonds**
1	**egg, beaten**
¼	**ounce (7 g) ground comfrey root**
1	**tablespoon (15 ml) honey**

To make:

Combine the almonds, egg, comfrey root, and honey, stirring with your hands or a wooden spoon. Refrigerate. (Of course, they didn't have refrigerators in the Middle Ages.)

To use:

1. Before bed, smooth this mixture over your hands and fingers and pull on either a pair of cotton gloves or old leather gloves. Follow this regimen for 7 nights.

2. Each morning, rinse your hands and the gloves and apply a skin lotion. After the nightly routine of the first week, cut back to a once-a-week schedule for a month, and then repeat this recipe only on a monthly basis.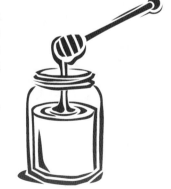

Caution: Internal use of comfrey is not recommended.

HAND AND NAIL BUTTER

Used daily or as necessary, this rich, moisturizing formula will soothe and soften dry, rough, chapped hands and cuticles. It smells like chocolate if left unscented.

2	tablespoons (30 ml) beeswax
2	tablespoons (30 ml) cocoa butter
4	tablespoons (60 ml) grapeseed or jojoba oil
1	tablespoon (15 ml) anhydrous lanolin
20	drops essential oil of rose, carrot seed, rosemary, geranium, or sandalwood (optional)

To make:

1. In the top part of a double boiler, warm all ingredients, except the essential oil, until the wax is melted.

2. Remove from heat and stir occasionally until almost cool.

3. Add the essential oil, if desired, stir again, and store in a cool, dark location. Use within 4 months.

To use:

Use approximately 1 teaspoon (5 ml) per application as a hand cream or nail and cuticle treatment. You can also use on your hands and feet as an overnight intensive treatment. Wear gloves or socks.

Note: This recipe may harden in cold water, but it will soften upon skin contact.

Nail and cuticle treatment: Soak clean hands in a bowl of warm water for 2 minutes. Pat dry. Apply a dab of the Hand and Nail Butter onto the base of each nail and massage in. Using a small piece of cotton flannel, gently push back your cuticles and lightly buff the nails with the cloth. Leaves fingertips soft and smooth.

Naturally shiny nail treatment: Apply the Hand and Nail Butter as directed in the nail and cuticle treatment above, but use a nail buffer to gently polish nails to a soft sheen. Don't rub so hard that your nails burn. Do this once a week.

MAKES APPROXIMATELY 25 TREATMENTS

Keeping Your Hands Looking Young

In many ways, our hands mirror and chronicle our life experiences. Abuse your hands, says Henrietta Spencer, and they will give away your most closely guarded secret — your age.

The age of your skin is partially determined by its content of water-soluble collagen. Collagen is a protein necessary for the formation of connective tissue, and it give skin its flexibility and capacity for absorbing moisture. When the skin becomes thin and less pliable, as it does through the aging process, collagen molecules have oxidized, formed bonds, cross-linked, and become stiffer and less able to swell or absorb moisture. Lines and wrinkles begin to appear. We notice these signs first on the face and neck and on the backs of the hands and arms. Over the years, these areas have been the most vulnerable to the cumulative effects of the sun's rays, which hasten the skin's cellular deterioration.

Skin Elasticity

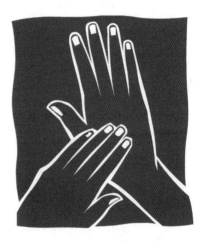

A gradual loss of skin elasticity is one of the hallmarks of the aging hand. New research on collagen and aging skin offers hope that we can delay deterioration in skin elasticity. Studies show that unrefined avocado oil inhibits the activity of the enzyme lysyl oxidase, which is partially responsible for cross-linking collagen. A simple avocado oil, as part of a natural, soluble collagen cream or added to your diet, just may help to slow the clock a bit. Avocado oil also has therapeutic value because it contains the vitamins A, D, and E; is easily absorbed into the skin, as it contains more than 20 percent essential fatty acids; accelerates healing of wounds and eczema; and offers some protection from the sun's damaging ultraviolet rays. If you think it's worth a try, take a look at the recipe on the next page.

AVOCADO SKIN CREAM

Oil-Soluble Ingredients

- ⅓ ounce (9 g) pure unbleached beeswax
- ¼ cup (60 ml) aromatic, soft green avocado oil
- 1 teaspoon (5 ml) calendula-infused oil (see recipe on facing page)
- 1½ teaspoons (7.5 ml) anhydrous lanolin; if you have a lanolin sensitivity, substitute cocoa butter or shea butter
- Contents of a soy lecithin capsule
- Contents of a vitamin E capsule

Water-Soluble Ingredients

- 1 tablespoon (15 ml) distilled water
- 1 teaspoon (5 ml) glycerin
- Pinch of borax
- Squeeze of strained lemon juice
- 10 drops essential oil of geranium, lavender, or patchouli

To make:

1. In the top part of a double boiler, combine the beeswax, avocado oil, calendula oil, and lanolin (or cocoa butter or shea butter). Heat, stirring constantly, until the beeswax is melted and the ingredients are well blended. Remove from heat.

2. In a separate pot, warm the distilled water, glycerin, borax, and lemon juice until all the dry ingredients are dissolved. Remove this mixture from the heat.

3. When the beeswax and oils mixture has cooled, stir in the contents of the lecithin capsule.

4. Slowly add half the water mixture to the beeswax mixture, stirring constantly.

5. Stir in the contents of the vitamin E capsule.

6. Slowly add the rest of the water and the essential oil, stirring constantly.

7. When the mixture resembles a mayonnaise texture, stop stirring and pour into a clean glass jar. Do not overmix or the cream will begin to separate. If the cream seems a bit runny, let it cool a minute, stir briefly, and then pour into a glass jar.

8. After it has completely cooled, cap tightly, label, and store in the refrigerator.

To use:

Whenever you notice your hands are looking dry, moisten each hand with water and pat dry. Massage in cream.

CALENDULA OIL

Calendula officinalis, *also known as pot marigold, is a sun-loving plant with yellow and deep orange flower heads. It contains both beta-carotene and vitamin C and is used in many skin-soothing preparations. It is particularly useful for chapped or cracked hands.*

1   cup (250 ml) dried calendula flowers
2   cups (500 ml) cold-pressed oil (olive, sweet almond, apricot, sesame, sunflower, or walnut)

To make:

1. Fill a clean glass jar to within an inch of the top with dried flowers. Then gently pack the flowers down with a spoon.

2. Slowly pour most of the oil into the jar, making sure that it completely covers the flowers. Stir gently with a non-metal utensil (such as a wooden chopstick) to release any trapped air bubbles. Then top off with the remaining oil and seal the jar with a lid or a double layer of cheesecloth secured with a rubber band.

3. Place the jar in a paper bag and set on a warm, sunny windowsill for 5 to 6 weeks. Turn the jar weekly and inspect for moisture. If there is moisture, open the jar, carefully wipe it off with a clean towel, and reseal.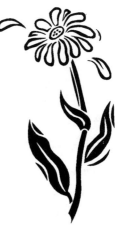

4. When the oil is a beautiful golden color, it is ready. Strain through cheesecloth to remove the flowers. Then strain again through a paper coffee filter to remove any smaller debris.

5. Pour the oil into clean jars, seal, and label. Store in a cool, dark location and use within 1 year.

Dry Skin

Dry skin can be a common problem as we age. The body's natural production of oil slows over the years. As our hormonal levels change — for women, as estrogen decreases — rough, dry skin develops because there is little hormonal stimulation to the sebaceous glands, which shrink in size and produce less oil. There is less of an oily surface, then, to attract moisture from the surrounding environment. Sun, wind, low humidity, artificial heating, air conditioning, air travel, and harsh detergent or antibacterial soaps further dehydrate and injure the skin. As we age, dry skin is most often noticeable on the backs of our hands and on our elbows.

For recipes to soothe and heal your dry skin, refer back to Moisturizers for Dry Skin (pages 12–17).

Age Spots

Age spots, sometimes incorrectly called "liver spots," usually show up on the backs of the hands and are caused by the cumulative effects of sunlight or chronic bruising of the skin. Unrefined avocado oil is a good remedy to try; it contains plant steroids, called sterolins, that have been found to diminish age spots and rebuild collagen. Use the oil in salads and rub it onto the backs of your hands. In addition, try the following recipe.

ONION JUICE AND VINEGAR WASH FOR AGE SPOTS

This is a traditional folk "cure" for age spots. It can also be used to prevent black-and-blue marks if rubbed on immediately after bruising the skin.

> **1 teaspoon (5 ml) freshly squeezed onion juice**
> **2 teaspoons (10 ml) organic apple cider vinegar**

To make:

Mix the onion juice with the vinegar

To use:

Pat this blend on the age spots on your hands at least once a day. Refrigerate any leftover mixture. The spots may begin to fade in a few weeks.

Resources

AromaTherapy Laboratories USA
800-722-4377
www.aromausa.com
Quality essential oils

Aubrey Organics
800-282-7394
www.aubrey-organics.com
Natural skin, hair, and body care

Dry Creek Herb Farm
888-489-8454
www.drycreekharbfarm.com
Wildcrafted bulk herbs and herbal products

Frontier Natural Products Co-op
800-669-3275
www.frontiercoop.com
Organic herbs, teas, and spices, plus essential oils

Gaia Herbs
800-831-7780
www.gaiaherbs.com
Extracts

Jean's Greens
518-479-0471
www.jeansgreens.com
Herbs and extracts

Liberty Natural Products
800-289-8427
www.libertynatural.com
Essential oils, extracts, herbs, and packaging supplies

Mountain Rose Herbs
800-879-3337
www.mountainroseherbs.com
Bulk organic herbs, teas, essential and carrier oils,
and packaging supplies

Other Storey Titles You Will Enjoy

The Aromatherapy Companion,
by Victoria H. Edwards.
The most comprehensive aromatherapy guide,
filled with profiles of essential oils and recipes
for beauty, health, and well-being.
288 pages. Paper. ISBN 978-1-58017-150-2.

The Herbal Home Remedy Book,
by Joyce A. Wardwell.
A wealth of herbal healing wisdom, with advice
on how to collect and store herbs, make remedies,
and stock a home herbal medicine chest.
176 pages. Paper. ISBN 978-1-58017-016-1.

The Herbal Home Spa: Naturally Refreshing Wraps,
Rubs, Lotions, Masks, Oils, and Scrubs,
by Greta Breedlove.
A collection of easy-to-create personal care
products that rival potions found at exclusive spas
and specialty shops.
208 pages. Paper. ISBN 978-1-58017-005-5.

Naturally Healthy Skin, by Stephanie Tourles.
A total reference about caring for all types of skin,
with recipes, techniques, and practical advice.
208 pages. Paper. ISBN 978-1-58017-130-4.

Organic Body Care Recipes, by Stephanie Tourles.
Homemade, herbal formulas for glowing skin, hair,
and nails, plus a vibrant self.
384 pages. Paper. ISBN 978-1-58017-676-7.

These and other books from Storey Publishing are available
wherever quality books are sold or by calling 1-800-441-5700.
Visit us at *www.storey.com.*